Emerging From the Cave

Emerging From the Cave

Surviving Graves' Disease

Celia Marie

Emerging From the Cave: Surviving Graves' Disease

This book is designed to provide accurate and authoritative information with regard to the subject matter covered. This information is given with the understanding that the author is not engaged in rendering legal, professional advice. Since the details of your situation are fact dependent, you should additionally seek the services of a competent professional.

Published in the United States of America

ISBN: 978-0-557-40911-2

1. Health & Fitness/Diseases/Immune System

2. Health & Fitness/Diseases/General

For Maria and my Papa

Maria: you are an amazing young woman and your strength, optimism and courage are an inspiration to me. You are the light of my life. I love you, Ri.

Papa: Richard Duron La Paglia, 1924-1979, you are my hero. I look at the brightest star and know it's you smiling on me and encouraging me each step of the way.

Contents

Acknowledgements

Katie Knapp edited my first book, *Life in the Cave: Overcoming Grave's Disease,* and I am forever grateful to her. She helped me to reach deeper and higher and was with me every step of the way as I strove to draw my readers into my thoughts and emotions during my experience of life in the cave.

Glynis Bonser has continued to be my special friend patiently listening, praying, crying and laughing with me on my journey of emerging from life in the cave. A friend loveth at all times. Proverbs 17:17

Deb Lowe has encouraged me since we were friends in second grade. She knows me better than most and continues to be a source of enthusiasm and joy! You have always been an inspiration to me, Deb.

Pat has provided the necessary medical insurance, paid for medical procedures, the doctors' visits, and prescriptions. Thank you.

Barb has rolled up her sleeves and not been afraid to help me during the most challenging of circumstances throughout our long friendship. I appreciate you, Barb.

My brother Pat was willing to come into the cave with me which helped me to not feel so alone in those early days. His visits in the beginning of this journey were my lifeline. The laughter we shared during the hours leading up to my surgery was exactly what I needed. Pat, you are the most amazing brother on the planet and I love you so much. Numbers 6:24-26 is one of my most favorite verses, too.

Eric has been a source of encouragement, strength and inspiration. Chase Cross. Gracias y bendiciones!

Introduction

You may have read my first book, *Life in the Cave: Overcoming Grave's Disease*, and have waited for months to learn of the details and outcome of my surgery. As promised, in this book I will begin with the first moments of the day of my surgery continuing my saga throughout the first year following my total thyroidectomy.

The two main reasons for choosing a total thyroidectomy are goiter (enlargement of the thyroid) and hyperthyroidism (overactive thyroid). In my case I had a huge goiter and severe hyperthyroidism. Two strikes against me. At one point my body was producing such an enormous amount of thyroxine that it could have kept fourteen people at a normal level. No wonder I couldn't relax, sit still, focus, and concentrate. My body was in a heightened state of activity all of the time. In addition to suffering from insomnia, I was a victim of nightmares, which caused an evening ritual of being perpetually wiped out, falling asleep and waking up in a total sweat from a panic attack. This cycle continued for over a year.

Due to the increasing size of my goiter, it began to press down on my windpipe, causing me to have difficulty breathing. My right lung was also affected and I was being treated for walking pneumonia. My skin was also becoming jaundiced as toxins flowed rampantly throughout my body. Sadly, I had the appearance of grave (no pun intended) illness because my vital organs were becoming poisoned. The combination of these medical issues presented a very serious challenge and it was the advanced stages of the goiter and hyperthyroidism that pointed to the only solution: a total thyroidectomy.

Although I did not want the total thyroidectomy I could no longer do the simplest of activities. Walking, standing, and sitting up and down were accomplished only with the greatest difficulty. In spite of these challenges, my surgeons were very optimistic that my body would tolerate the surgery well and heal properly. I had to trust their expertise and professional opinion. Their enthusiasm and confidence provided the glimmer of hope that I needed.

At this point I'd like to list the symptoms of Graves' disease. They include anxiety, brittle hair, fatigue, frequent bowel movements, goiter, increase in perspiration, insomnia, irritability, rapid/irregular heartbeat, sensitivity to heat, and weight loss. Further, Graves' Opthalmopathy and Graves' Dermopathy are two conditions that Graves' disease patients may experience. The symptoms of Graves' Opthalmopathy are excessive tearing (sensation of grit or sand in either/both eyes), reddened/inflamed eyes, widening of the space between eyelids, swelling of the lids and tissues around the eyes, and light sensitivity. My condition has definitely improved since my total thyroidectomy but I still experience the tearing, reddened eyes and light sensitivity. The symptoms of Graves' dermopathy are reddening/swelling of the skin, often on shins and top of feet. It has been two years since my surgery and I have seen little improvement and healing of my shins and top of my feet. I will share with you my personal experiences with each of these symptoms. Every case is unique, though, and you or your loved one may not have each of these symptoms.

Looking back it was the spring of 2006 that finally yielded all of the above symptoms. The anxiety was noticeable to others by then. For example, my boss walked into my classroom and said, "Celia, you are anxious, aren't you?" In addition, I was fatigued to the point of falling asleep at work as Tiffany, my outgoing and cheerful student, would giggle shouting "teacher, wake up!", a coworker commented and teased me about my frequent trips to the bathroom, and two coworkers told me a few times that my neck area looked swollen.

Compliments on my much slimmer body began during the summer of 2005 and continued through the spring of 2006. Even though it was exciting to receive praise for the huge amount, nearly sixty pounds, of weight loss it was a negative symptom because my body was in an acute hyperactive state of metabolism. My hair began falling out in March of 2006, too. I was also experiencing severe sensitivity to heat and, beginning as early as February, I wore shorts and short sleeve tops. The inability to sleep at night was becoming more frequent. Crankiness might as well have been my middle name, along with the continual rapid heartbeat which was alarming to me. All of these symptoms were an indication of Graves' disease. I was formally diagnosed with Graves' disease and hyperthyroidism during September of 2006.

The purpose of writing my first book was to reach out to that one person who knew that something was dreadfully wrong with their body but was paralyzed with fear and chose not to seek medical attention. I wanted to share how the fear that gripped me made it much more difficult for my body to withstand and heal from this autoimmune disorder. My daughter, my husband, my family members and close friends, along with my coworkers, were all negatively affected by my decision to not seek early medical intervention. I know full well how fear can totally grip and paralyze you and I also know what it's like to see hurt, despair and fear affect those closest to you because you are stuck in a moment you can't find a way to get out of.

My main purpose in writing *Emerging From the Cave* is to share with you the joys and disappointments of the outcome of my total thyroidectomy and reveal how my life has continued to change in the past two years. I hope that medical professionals (doctors, nurses, phlebotomists, ultrasound technicians, thyroid scan uptake technicians, x-ray technicians, nursing students, surgeons, endocrinologists and autoimmune disorder researchers) will find this book helpful in seeing the humanity of the Graves' disease patient and I pray that you, the Graves' disease patient or loved one, will find encouragement and hope within the pages of this book you are reading in your hands, on your wireless device or perhaps even listening to via audio book as you drive.

Graves' disease is a treatable but not curable autoimmune disease. At the time of this writing there is still no cure for Graves' disease. I hope that I will be living when a cure is found. I do not wish this disease upon anyone because this is a life altering condition that affects all facets of your being. I believe that we all have four important components in our being: physical, mental, emotional and spiritual. Graves' disease affects each of these areas. I have found that when I nurture all of these areas I am surviving and overcoming Graves' disease.

If you have read *Life in the Cave Overcoming Grave's Disease* you will know that my spiritual being was what I tapped into when I had hit rock bottom with no place to go but up. Although this book will focus more on physical, mental and emotional areas I want to share with you that prayer and scripture reading continue to be a daily part of my life. I do believe in physical healing although I have not yet been fully healed of Graves' disease. If you believe in the power of prayer, please join me in praying that a cure for Graves' disease is found.

I want to publicly thank Dr. Richard Harding and Dr. Bryce, my amazing thyroidectomy surgeons and the beautiful nurse of color who gently, carefully took care of me during my first twelve hours after surgery and treated me with the utmost respect and dignity as my body came out of the anesthesia. I am so sorry that I do not remember your name but you are my hero. I hope that you will always be successful in your nursing career. I salute you.

I would also like to salute the small population (mostly women) who daily battle Graves' disease. A portion of the proceeds of this book goes to the National Graves' Disease Foundation located in Buffalo, New York. It is my deepest desire that you will receive information that will challenge you to learn even more about Graves' disease and join us in achieving Graves' disease awareness in our homes, communities, states and the world.

Celia Marie

May 2010

Chapter One
February 25, 2008

It was a beautiful morning and the sun shone brightly. The air was slightly chilly, yet pleasant. I lay peacefully in bed for a moment before I remembered that this was the day I was to go in for my total thyroidectomy. I immediately began to fight waves of panic as my mind began racing with the thought of what if I die during surgery? I attempted to calm myself down with positive thoughts and thankfulness that I had two experienced surgeons whom I trusted performing my surgery. Now that I was calm I leaned over to say good morning to our Australian Cattle Dog, Boomer, who was lying peacefully on his very own leather bed right beside me.

I walked into Maria's bedroom and gently woke up my daughter, gave her a kiss and told her that I loved her. I reminded her that today was my surgery and we needed to get ready to go to the hospital. Glynis (my longtime friend of twenty-one years) was driving over to meet us and would follow us to the hospital. I had packed my overnight bag the night before and included my CD player along with my *Best of Sixpence None the Richer* CD. We put my belongings in the car and waited for Glynis to arrive. While we were waiting, I said goodbye to Boomer, Jade (my lynx point Siamese cat) and Snickers (my daughter's bunny rabbit). Tears were in my eyes and a huge lump was in my throat as I hugged each of them. They were more than pets—they were family.

Glynis drove up right on time and after we greeted each other with hugs, exchanged a little bit of small talk and then decided which route was best to take, we all got into our separate cars and drove to Banner Thunderbird hospital in Glendale, AZ. We went to the admitting area and waited about ten minutes before I met with a hospital staff person who asked me to provide personal information along with a copy of my will. I signed several documents and paid hundreds of dollars for my hospital stay co-pay. It seems like it took around twenty minutes for the complete admitting process and then we walked to the waiting room area. I was surprised that the nurse called me in to the pre-op room within less than five minutes after arriving.

Much to my disappointment, no one was allowed to come in with me while I waited as they prepared the room for me. I sat in a chair for at least fifteen minutes before the nurse actually called me into my pre-op room. I was instructed to undress and put on a hospital gown as the medical assistant closed the curtain.

Several minutes later my nurse asked me, through the closed curtain, if I needed any help and I replied "yes, I do." She opened the curtain and when I turned around I realized that she was Emily, the mom of one of my students. I was surprised and delighted to discover that Emily was going to be my nurse. It is such a small world.

As Emily and I chatted about Claire I began to relax. I asked to see a picture of Claire and Emily obliged. It had been two years since I had seen Claire or Emily. While Emily wrote down my vitals I looked at the walls of my room. It was decorated in a beach theme. I was so humbled that God even orchestrated the smallest of things to make me comfortable. During college I loved surfing; in fact, my bedroom was decorated with a surfer's beach theme. I was extremely thankful to God for arranging this beach-themed hospital room for me because it was familiar, comforting and helped me to relax.

After I settled in, Maria and Glynis came to visit me. About an hour later my brother, Pat, stopped by. We talked and laughed a lot. We had always gotten along well together and this day was no different. After he left Maria and Glynis came back in to sit with me again. My surgery was scheduled for 1:00 but around 12:30 a new nurse (Emily's shift had recently ended) informed me that Dr. Harding and Dr. Bryce were running behind schedule.

An x-ray was ordered for my right lung because I was having breathing complications. After the x-ray was performed we waited and waited for the results. Maria and Glynis decided to get lunch at the hospital cafeteria and while they were eating my brother came back in to see me. The results of the lung x-ray were not good. Dr. Harding wanted to postpone the surgery for a few more hours to see if my lung would improve.

Truthfully, I was hoping that Dr. Harding would decide I was too ill and weak to perform the surgery. We waited until around 3:00 pm before another x-ray of my lung was taken. Two hours later Dr. Harding came in to discuss the results with me. He said that my lung was doing marginally better but because my goiter was huge it was causing my trachea area to collapse which explained why I was having extreme difficulty breathing along with the complications of my right lung. My skin also appeared jaundiced. Dr. Harding said that if he didn't perform the surgery that day he was uncertain if I would pull through because I was critically ill. He decided that he and Dr. Bryce would perform my total thyroidectomy at 6:00 pm. My surgery would be their last surgery of the day.

A few minutes before my surgery, Pat (Maria's dad), came in to see me for about five minutes. After he left, Maria and Glynis stayed with me until the nurse placed the anesthesia in my I.V. Within approximately five minutes after administering the anesthesia, the nurse wheeled me out of my pre-op room as I waved goodbye to Maria and Glynis, telling Maria that I loved her.

Chapter Two
February 26, 2008

After telling Maria that I loved her as the nurse was wheeling me out of my pre-op room, my next thought was that I must have survived the surgery because I was awake. (Actually, nine hours had passed since I had fallen asleep). Praise God, I'm going to see Maria grow up after all! I was so thankful to God for allowing me to survive the surgery as tears welled up in my eyes. I looked at the clock and it was around 3:00 am.

Huge waves of nausea overtook me while I was looking at the clock and I began to vomit everywhere. I was so humiliated and embarrassed. I tried to apologize to the nurse but could barely speak. I didn't realize yet that a hose was crammed down deep into my throat and trachea area. I continued to vomit and began to cry because I felt ashamed about being violently ill in front of the nurse. She assured me that there was no need to apologize. I fell asleep after that.

When I woke up I was staring at a hole in the wall. All of the meds I was taking made me feel groggy, nauseated, and like I was in a fog. I couldn't even speak above a whisper. I slowly realized that I was hooked up to several monitors along with oxygen tubes in my nostrils. It was very uncomfortable to be limited in mobility because of all of the various tubes and hoses connected to my body and a myriad of machines. I fell asleep again. Someone woke me up to tell me that they needed to take an x-ray of my right lung. I tried to move as best as I could but I was weak and miserable. I then fell back asleep.

The next time I woke up Maria and Pat were coming into my ICU room. Maria looked terribly frightened to see all of the hoses and tubes connected to me. My eyes were still bulging and I had a huge gauze bandage covering my neck area; two drains had also been placed in my neck where the goiter had been removed. I truly believed that I must have looked like an alien. Later, Pat told me that I looked dreadful; even the nurses seemed appalled at my appearance but these ICU nurses were always kind, gentle and respectful towards me. Pat described me as a holocaust survivor which meant that even though I was technically alive, I looked dead.

I was overjoyed to see Maria but equally sobered and concerned to see her frightened expression at my appearance. She slowly walked over to me and offered me a beautiful, soft, white polar bear that I could hold on to for comfort. Maria is   exceptionally sweet and thoughtful. I was extremely proud of my kind and loving daughter. She also brought me a get well card with a picture of a puppy with a band-aid on his forehead. The card was "signed" by all of our pets along with Maria and Pat. I smiled and tried to laugh as I read the card. I still have that card on my dresser as a reminder of the love that surrounded me the morning after my surgery and still does.

I drifted in and out of sleep. I asked Maria if we were waiting for me to go in for my surgery and she replied, "No, Mom, they did your surgery yesterday." I was understandably confused from all of the meds they were giving me and also drained from the physical trauma that my body underwent during my total thyroidectomy.

After the next round of meds, Glynis came to see me for a few minutes before she drove back to California. I was sad to see her leave because I appreciated her for taking time out of her busy schedule to be with Maria during my surgery and I also enjoyed her company. We have always found something to laugh about even in the most stressful situations. This hospital scenario was no different.

About an hour after Glynis left, my brother Pat came to see me. He looked awfully concerned when he saw me for the first time after my surgery. It was quite humiliating to have my loved ones see me looking horrible but I was exceedingly thankful that they were there with me. I couldn't speak to them very well because my vocal chords were very sore from the surgery and the trachea tube was jabbed down my throat. I appreciated seeing their faces with their love shining in their eyes for me.

I drifted in and out of sleep for the rest of the day. Maria and Pat came back to visit me during the evening hours. I discovered that there were even IVs in my feet and I was also hooked up to a catheter. All of this was so humiliating to me. My ICU nurse was extremely kind and respectful towards me. She made sure to keep me cleaned up (I was still vomiting a lot). She smelled so nice. I was exceedingly blessed to have her as my nurse during the first day after surgery and I sadly whispered goodbye when her shift ended.

After meeting my evening nurse I quickly discovered that she was very efficient and kind as she asked me what she could do to make me comfortable. Earlier in the day I had decided that I no longer wanted to be in ICU and requested to be moved to a private room several times during the day but my surgeons and pulmonary doctor didn't believe I was strong enough. Being the tenacious person that I am, I asked my new nurse if I could be moved to a private room and she told me that she would find out. My vitals were taken and after about an hour and a half she came back and said that a private room was being prepared for me. I was relieved and thankful. She removed my catheter and helped me into the restroom.

While I was in the restroom a thin pinkish bloody fluid began leaking from the huge gauze bandage in my neck area. I was alarmed as I pushed the emergency button for the nurse. She helped me get all cleaned up. Once again I was humiliated to be in this offensive condition. I apologized to her (although it was very difficult for me to speak) for the mess and she graciously said that no apology was necessary. She then helped me get seated in the chair because I didn't want to lie down in the bed as I waited for the wheelchair to be delivered to my ICU room in order to be transported to my private room.

Around 10pm I rode in the wheelchair to my new room. My nurse was in her early 20s and she commented on my daughter's Christy Miller book that was placed on the nightstand. She went on to say that she liked the music I was playing. I told her that the band was *Sixpence None the Richer* and she commented that she had heard of them and liked them. She then asked me if I wanted morphine for the pain and I hastily and emphatically replied "no." I was scared to take morphine because I saw how it had negatively affected Carole, my mother-in-law, when she was administered it during her last stage of lung cancer.

At 10:30 pm I asked the young nurse if Maria could spend the night with me and she said that Maria was not old enough to stay. I was extremely disappointed as I hugged Maria good night telling her I loved her. Maria and I have always been close and I didn't want to spend the night by myself in my private room. I was scared that something could go wrong and I wanted Maria with me as much as possible. I waved goodnight to her and we signed "I love you" to each other as she walked out of the hospital room. I then cried and looked at her Christy Miller book on my nightstand while I listened to Leigh Bingham Nash's soothing voice sing "Trust in the Lord" along with the brilliant talents of the *Sixpence None the Richer* musicians in the background.

When my nurse came in to check on me I asked her if she would help me as I tried to prop my neck area/head on the bed because there was no way that I could lie flat. It was very difficult to get in and out of the hospital bed and my incision area continued to ooze the thin pinkish bloody fluid. My nurse gave me a new hospital gown because the fluid kept leaking onto my gown. After I finally got settled in my new room I tried to go to sleep. Impossible. I didn't like to be alone and I was still in pain from the surgery feeling horrible and blurry from all of the meds that I was taking.

Chapter Three
February 27, 2008

I finally dozed off and was awakened by someone wanting to take another x-ray of my lung. Once again it took me awhile to drift off to sleep and then another young nurse came in to take my vitals. Lovely. It was now 3:00 am and I didn't want to be in the hospital anymore. I missed Maria, Boomer, Snickers and Jade. I couldn't sleep. It was just too noisy in the hospital.

Around 6:00 am Dr. Bryce (one of my surgeons) came in to see how I was doing. He had also checked on me while I was in ICU. He talked to me for quite a while and told me that I had given him and Dr. Harding (my primary surgeon) a run for their money as my surgery was the second liveliest/bloodiest that Dr. Harding had ever performed but they were up for it and I was up for it. He went on to say that they were able to remove all of the goiter and it was about three times the size of a healthy thyroid—no wonder I was ill and having such difficulty breathing.

Dr. Bryce then proceeded to remove the drains from my neck and I almost passed out when I saw how long the tubes were that had been inside my neck. His next step was to put a clean gauze bandage over my incision. He told me to wash the area with antibacterial soap daily. At the time I had no idea how hideous I still looked and now I have the utmost respect for him because he treated me with a great amount of respect and concern while sitting on the edge of my hospital bed just hours after my surgery. You see, my eyes were terribly swollen, red and watery. My face was very puffy. I had a huge bandage over my neck area which concealed a fresh three and a half inch incision that was oozing a thin, pinkish liquid. Within this incision area the surgeons inserted two drains. I had repeatedly vomited after my total thyroidectomy and hadn't been able to brush my teeth. I also hadn't been given the opportunity to have my hair brushed. Although I'm certain I looked exceedingly ugly, we chatted (I mostly listened because I could only speak in a whisper) for a few minutes more before he told me that he would come back and check on me. After Dr. Bryce left, my pulmonary specialist came in to see how I was doing. He informed me that he had been monitoring my lungs hours before my surgery (especially the right one) and that during surgery the right lung had completely shut down. He went on to say that he was going to continue to monitor it throughout the day. About an hour after he left, Maria and Pat came to visit. Pat stayed for a few minutes and then informed me that was going to show properties (he's a realtor) to one of his clients. Maria stayed with me all day and I was thankful to have her with me. Maria asked me if I needed anything as she held my hand. She is such a joy to be with and I enjoy her cheerful and easygoing personality. She was going to be twelve years old within a few weeks time and I was very proud of the way that she was handling my surgery and hospital stay.

I was also thankful that my friend Glynis came out from San Diego to be with Maria during my surgery. I asked Glynis to share her perspective on the waiting room along with the next morning after my surgery and this is what she had to say.

"Maria and I waved goodbye to Celia as she was rolled out of the prep room and taken to the operating room. I breathed another prayer for her, but in my heart knew that she was going to come through this. As we walked down the hall I put my arm around Maria's shoulders and gave her a little hug.

In the waiting room Maria was kept occupied with the few toys she had brought with her, but the pillow and the blanket are what gave her comfort. She and her dad Pat took a few walks outside of the room and I bought her some candy out of the machine that was conveniently located nearby.

Celia's brother Pat was there and the two of us had some serious dialogue about his baby sister. As I saw the concern in his eyes and heard the worry in his voice, it dawned on me how much he truly loved and cared for Celia Marie. It touched my heart.

As the time marched on I kept praying for Celia, and the men kept checking to see if the surgeons were to come out and talk to us soon. Finally, someone came and got us and took us to an area just outside the double swinging doors where the doctors would emerge and give us the news about Celia.

The surgeons came out and we anxiously listened to every word. Celia was in recovery and doing fine! Dr. Harding smiled victoriously and chuckled in disbelief when he told us that Celia's was the bloodiest thyroid surgery he had ever done and that he had been doing this for thirteen years. He told us that the goiter was huge and a bleeder. I prayed within myself thanking our loving Heavenly Father for the success of the surgery and petitioning Him for Celia's recovery.

With lighter hearts we headed to the parking lot. Maria and her dad separated from Pat and me as we continued to go towards our cars. Pat was so relieved that his sister was doing okay and was telling me how special and beautiful Celia was.

The next morning I came by to see Celia before I headed back home to San Diego. I walked into her ICU room and there she lay weak, sick and miserable with tubes and machines all around her. My heart went out to her. She looked like she hurt on every inch of her body. Her neck was so bandaged up that it looked as if she couldn't move it. Her eyes were swollen and watery and it was all she could do to get out a whisper. I could tell that it hurt her to talk. Celia's husband and daughter were there with her so I didn't stay long. I knew she needed to rest so I prayed with her and assured her that although she had a long road ahead of her, she was going to be okay and would get better." Thank you, Glynis, for sharing your perspective with us.

Around 11:00 am I desperately wanted to leave the hospital and I asked the nurse if I could be discharged. She came back to say, "No, your levels aren't stable enough to be released." I was very disappointed. A few hours later I again asked if I could leave. She said that she would contact my surgeons to see if it could be arranged. My levels had finally improved enough and they agreed to release me on the condition that I would faithfully take calcium pills because my calcium level was borderline. I promised that I would.

I asked if I could take a shower and the nurse brought me shampoo, soap, a towel and washcloth. It was one of the most challenging showers that I have ever taken in my life because I had to be very careful around the incision area. I was still very weak. Once I finished my shower and got dressed I looked in the mirror. I looked repulsive. My eyes were still bulging. My face was very puffy and red. The gauze over my neck area looked awful. I started to cry. I thought that my appearance would improve once I had the surgery. In actuality, I looked worse than I did before the surgery. I was extremely disappointed and so very tired of being ugly.

Around 3:00 pm I was relieved when the nurse brought my discharge papers for me to sign. In less than a half-hour I was in the car and heading home. It was a record-breaking heat day in the 90s and it was very hot in the car. I didn't care, though, because I was out of that noisy hospital.

Chapter Four
Home at Last

I slowly and carefully got out of the car with Maria's help and walked to the door. I don't remember who unlocked the door but I saw Boomer through the glass windows of the French door waiting on the other side. When I opened the door he greeted me with a friendly bark then he started whimpering and I started crying while I attempted to hug him. We were locked in this moment of time completely unaware of anything else but each other. I realized then how much Boomer loved me and how much I loved him. From that moment on, Boomer has been my greatest protector and companion. Maria and Pat said that he continually looked for me all throughout the house during my hospital stay. I never realized the special bond that Boomer and I had formed until we were separated. Boomer is my forever friend. I was so thankful to be reunited with him and grateful to be home.

I walked slowly into the kitchen with Boomer by my side. He wanted to be right beside me and that comforted me. It seemed so surreal to be at home. I was still pumped up with all of the meds given to me at the hospital and I felt like I was having some out-of-body experience as I looked around like I was seeing all of my familiar surroundings for the first time through another person's eyes.

As I walked down the hallway to my bedroom my eyes welled up with tears. The best way I can describe what I was feeling is to compare it with the way a runner may feel when participating in a very challenging marathon. The runner is halfway through the marathon and doesn't want to turn back now but is weary and knows he's only halfway there. I had hoped to come home with normal looking eyes, a thinner face, healthy looking hair and a slimmer body. Instead I was in physical pain from the incision, along with emotional pain from my unrealistic expectations. I was angry that my life wasn't going to ever be the way it was before this ominous autoimmune disease attacked my body.

Now that I was in my bedroom I tried to get into bed but it was such a challenging task. I had propped up several pillows to elevate my head because there was no way that I could lay down flat. The incision in my neck area was larger than my surgeons anticipated and they explained that they had to cut further into my muscle tissue due to the size of the goiter. As a result, the muscles in my neck and shoulder area were very sore. I could barely move my neck side to side without experiencing a great deal of pain. I finally got settled in and fell asleep for a few hours. I woke up and slowly walked to the family room while Boomer followed closely behind me. I sat in the oversized leather chair and wished that the physical pain in my neck area would just go away. It didn't. I started having that bizarre out-of-body sensation all over again but because the pain was so intense I found myself compelled to take another pain pill. Throughout the night I slept, woke up, dozed, got up to take some more meds and then fell back into a troubled sleep.

I don't remember what time I woke up the next morning. But I do know that even though my first full day home from the hospital was a blur it was good to be home. I saw Snickers for the first time and he seemed happy to see me, too. I smiled as I reached down to pet him. I was immediately overwhelmed with intense pain. It hurt to bend down. I still hadn't seen Jade and was eager to talk to her and pet her soft fur.

Throughout the day Maria asked me if I needed anything. She was a great help to me with whatever task I was unable to do. After I drifted in and out of sleep during the day, I needed to change my gauze dressing. That proved to be a daunting task as I tried to put the sterile gauze square on top of the incision then attempted to cut the tape to secure the gauze dressing with only one hand while the other held up the sterile gauze square. Frustrating.

The day consisted of taking meds at assigned times and trying to eat. My trachea area was incredibly sore from the trachea tube. Eating pudding was painful and drinking liquid was too. The calcium pills that I had been prescribed were huge and it hurt to swallow them. The effects that the trachea tube had left on my throat and windpipe area irritated me. I didn't like the nausea I was experiencing. I had to remind myself to be grateful that the surgery was behind me and better days were ahead of me.

It continued to be a challenge to get in and out of bed but I still slept a lot. At bedtime I decided to try to sleep in the oversized leather chair in the family room. Boomer joined me by sleeping on the leather love seat beside me. After waking up several times that night I slowly walked back to the bedroom and propped up the pillows and got into bed. I awoke about an hour later with a severe panic attack. I decided right then and there to stop taking the pain pill. I hated having panic attacks. I still felt like an alien and was tired of having the out-of-body sensation feelings. I never took a pain pill after that night.

Chapter Five
Hypothyroidism

The first week home proved to be more challenging than I had anticipated. As I gazed at my reflection in the mirror after I had taken my shower I gasped at the huge bruises on my chest area, my shoulders and my upper arms. I looked like I was pummeled badly in a street fight and I had lost. I wondered if perhaps I flatlined during surgery.

I was irritated that I was not getting stronger by now and I could barely talk above a whisper. It literally hurt to try to project my voice. I could not talk loud enough to have a conversation on the phone and I was still too weak to get on the internet to read e-mails and go on MySpace to communicate with family and friends. Totally frustrating.

Finally, on the fourth day after my surgery, I was strong enough to check my e-mails. I had received hundreds and I found it to be too daunting to read through them all. I scanned through them and answered the ones from family and close friends. I also tried to talk on the phone but could only talk for a couple of minutes because it hurt my vocal chords to speak. At least I could communicate through e-mail and MySpace so that was encouraging.

On Tuesday at 9:00 am I met with Dr. Harding for my complimentary post-op consultation. Dr. Harding was optimistic, enthusiastic and encouraging as he talked to me while examining my neck area. He asked me to repeat vowel sounds after him and observed that I was having difficulty sounding out the vowels. Although I was concerned about this struggle he reassured me that my vocal chords were healing and I would, in time, master the correct pronunciation of the vowels.

Dr. Harding went on to share with me the test results were in and said the words I had been praying to hear since 2006: "Celia, there was not a bit of cancer in your goiter". He went on to say "and we meticulously removed and scraped the entire goiter out." Tears welled up in my eyes as I exclaimed, "Praise God, thank you Dr. Harding!" I saw the joy in his eyes and the sense of accomplishment on his face that he was satisfied with a job well done. As I quickly looked over at Maria to see her response to the good news she looked relieved, excited and had a tear in her eye as it dawned on her that her mother was not going to die from thyroid cancer.

Our drive home was filled with shouts of "awesome" and "thank you, Jesus" in the car as we travelled from downtown Phoenix back to Glendale. I don't think I ever stopped praising God all the way home. For two years I had been paralyzed with fear that I had thyroid cancer and to have that burden which weighed a million tons lifted off of me was totally phenomenal. I wish I could articulate exactly what this freedom from the fear of cancer meant to me. The chains from the mental and emotional oppression and torment were released and the shackles from the paralysis of fear were broken off of my feet. It also brought me great joy to see the change of countenance in Maria. She lifted her face upward, squared her shoulders back in confidence and walked with a lighter step. The good news that I had not a bit of cancer was also a testimony of the power of prayer and faith to Maria and me.

I reflected back to my meetings with Dr. Duick (my second endocrinologist) and Dr. Harding and they both concurred that without a thyroid my body would go hypothyroid. I was praying that the Lord would spare me and heal my body from having to experience hypothyroidism. He had other plans for me, though.

I wasn't looking forward to the eleven symptoms of hypothyroidism which are brittle hair, depression, dry skin, elevated blood cholesterol level, fatigue, increased sensitivity to cold, muscle aches, tenderness, stiffness, muscle weakness, puffy face, sluggishness, and weight gain.

I did not experience the above symptoms the minute my thyroid was removed. Over time, though, I began to have symptoms of hypothyroidism and now, two years later, I have all of the hypothyroidism symptoms. Muscle aches, tenderness, stiffness and weakness occurred almost immediately following the surgery.

The muscle aches were to the level of pain that I would cry out in misery. I would cry because my muscles would cramp up so bad. The pain was unbearable and I could not move the muscle involved. This could occur in any muscle at any time. The most prevalent area, though, was the back of my legs, my feet and my toes. I would also experience horrific muscle cramps in my chest cavity area and the back of my neck. I never knew when the muscle cramps were going to start and I had no way to prepare for them. Sometimes they would strike at the grocery store, at home, at the movies or at church. It was frightening when they would suddenly come upon me in the shower. I had to constantly take extra precautions in the shower for fear that I would fall and strike my head during the fall.

Sluggishness was another symptom I faced immediately after my surgery. I kept complaining to my endocrinologist about the sluggishness and he finally prescribed Cytomel in July of 2008. Two years later I am still taking Cytomel daily. Cytomel is a synthetic form of a natural thyroid hormone. I am now hypothyroid because I no longer have a thyroid and the Synthroid (thyroid hormone drug) isn't producing enough of the thyroid hormone that my body needs to function. Most patients who undergo a thyroidectomy will wind up being hypothyroid after their thyroid has been surgically removed.

Many months following the total thyroidectomy I noticed my hair beginning to grow back and although I was elated to have hair again I was disappointed that my hair was growing back thin and brittle. My hair used to be thick and wavy. To this day my hair is thin and brittle. It is just another reality that I've had to accept while surviving Graves' disease. While my hair was falling out I would wear fashionable hats. It was fun going to the department stores to try on hats. I still have the hats and they are a reminder of how far I've come.

In 2009 I began a naturopathic approach to dealing with elevated cholesterol levels and increased insulin levels. I began cardio and strength training which consisted of an urban belly dance workout and a George Foreman regimen. I stopped drinking caffeinated beverages and eliminated soda. I started eating more servings of fresh, steamed veggies and added freshly squeezed lemon to my water. My goal was to drink 64 ounces of water daily. I still incorporate all of these natural remedies in my daily activities. Unfortunately in February of 2010, despite the naturopathic therapy, my cholesterol and insulin levels were still too high so my doctor prescribed Crestor (synthetic lipid-lowering agent) and Metformin (antihyperglycemic agent). It is now June of 2010 and I am still taking these meds daily in addition to the naturopathic regimen which also consists of aromatherapy.

Dry skin has been a huge issue for me, especially in my lower legs and feet. I have never had the most attractive feet and it has been embarrassing to have them look even worse with the acute dry skin problem. I use Eucerin Dry Skin Therapy Everyday Protection Body Lotion with SPF15 and this product is very effective in moisturizing and protecting my skin.

My face and neck area continues to be combination (normal/oily) along with myxedema prominent on both my left and right cheeks which causes redness. I have found that Clinique Dramatically Different Moisturizing Lotion has worked wonders on my facial skin. I have not found a remedy for my puffy face, though, much to my chagrin.

I noticed the increased sensitivity to cold during 2009. When I was hyperthyroid I would wear shorts and sleeveless tops in the winter but now I wear sweaters and jeans while everyone else is sporting shorts and sleeveless tops!

Because I already battled depression with the Graves' disease and hyperthyroidism I don't believe that going hypothyroid impacted me that much. Whenever I would feel the depression coming on I would remind myself how much I really believe that laughter is one of the best ways to combat depression. I enjoy comedies and humorous books. I also enjoy laughing with Maria and my close friends Glynis and Barb.

When I was in college one of my psychology professors shared that he conducted a study on humor therapy and the results of his study revealed that humor is conducive to evoking a happier and more positive sense of wellbeing. If you are struggling with depression I highly recommend that you read humorous books, watch comedies, listen to upbeat music and look at the cup half full as often as possible. An attitude of gratitude is very important. Make a list of everything that you are thankful for and refer to your list daily. Positive thoughts are more powerful than negativity. A thankful heart is a happy heart. Laughter, smiles and positive thoughts produce endorphins which uplift your mood.

Weight gain hasn't affected me much since I have become hypothyroid. What I deal with now is metabolism issues. Because my insulin production is way off my metabolism is practically non-existent. No how matter how much I workout and reduce calories I am unable to lose weight. This metabolism malady is my Waterloo. I have shared my concerns with my doctor and he stated that the Metformin should help jump-start my metabolism. It's been two months since I've been on Metformin and I've yet to see even one ounce of weight loss.

Each of us is different and if you've been diagnosed with Hypothyroidism you may not have all of the symptoms I've listed and discussed. In most situations these symptoms can be effectively treated. I feel compelled to point out that only you truly know your body and if you are unhappy with the results of the medication your doctor has prescribed for you make sure you speak up. It doesn't matter what the test results indicate. If you're not feeling right you may need to get your dosage adjusted. You may even have to find another doctor who will listen to your concerns. Look out for yourself because you're the only one who knows exactly how you are doing.

Chapter Six
Social Security Disability Process

You may be experiencing severe stress because of a lack of income. A possible income solution available to you if you are unable to work is social security disability. There are three stages of the social security disability process. They are application, decision, and appeals process. Two optional and additional steps are retaining legal counsel and the appeals decision. This was indeed one of the most stressful and grievous issues of my battle with Graves' disease and hyperthyroidism.

I turned in my resignation on June 9, 2006 and was too fatigued to even look for a part-time job. It was now November of 2006 and we were beginning to feel the financial crunch of being a one income family. During a phone conversation my friend Barb suggested that I consider filing for social security disability. I thanked her for the suggestion and told her that I would think about it. I really didn't want to go this route but I was in such bad, physical shape that this looked like my only option.

I went online to discover how to start the whole social security disability process. Please keep in mind that I was in an acute state of confusion and lack of focus was an everyday occurrence. It took everything I had to read the instructions on how to apply for disability. It literally took hours for me to comprehend what I was supposed to do. I had to take frequent breaks because my eyes teared up often as I attempted to read the words on the computer screen. Finally, on November 5, 2006, with much trepidation, I was ready to begin filing for social security disability. I applied online. They demanded a plethora of information. I struggled to gather the required tax information, job history, medical history and a myriad of other information to complete the online application. Eight hours later I was finished but the utter frustration of the process left me in tears and total exhaustion.

The next step was to find out if the social security administration received my online application. I received an e-mail that it was indeed received. Great, I thought. I prayed that it would not take long to receive my social security disability benefit payments. I didn't think much about it during the holidays because I was busy with the Radioactive Iodine (RAI) therapy on November 29, 2006, focusing on the holiday season and anticipating a positive outcome, dreaming of no more bulging eyes, no more rapid heartbeat, no more anxiety, no more insomnia and returning to my normal self.

Within two weeks of filing, I received a big manila envelope from social security instructing me to fill out the enclosed paperwork which needed to be sent to each doctor and medical provider who was involved in my case. It took several hours to complete the paperwork as it required that I list each provider involved and look up their mailing address, phone number, and give detailed information of the service that each provided. In mid-January I e-mailed Pam, my social security contact, and she confirmed that my file was being looked at but would take a few more weeks before a decision was made.

It was now March of 2007 but I received no news of a decision about my case. Nine months of being a single income family was definitely taking its toll. Thankfully we did not have car payments to make but we had real estate broker's fees that needed to be paid along with all of the realtor fees due (national, state, MLS, Supra realtor fees). It upset me that we had to have a more toned-down birthday party for my daughter (her birthday is March 13) but she didn't complain.

The months went by and in May of 2007 I spoke to a Social Security Administration worker who informed me that he needed documentation from one of my doctors who had never responded to my original request for a doctor's report. I asked if this would have a negative effect on my case and he stated that it was almost the cut-off date for a decision to be made and he needed the documentation immediately.

My brother, Dan, e-mailed me frequently and asked how my social security application was coming along. As I shared with him my frustrations he responded that he and Pamelia (his wife) would continue to pray for me. He encouraged me to keep trusting the Lord.

Finally, during the month of June, I received the much-anticipated letter from social security. I anxiously opened the letter looking forward to a positive response. I was utterly disappointed to read that my request had been denied. The letter revealed that I could appeal the decision and gave instructions on how to begin the appeals process. I had no other choice but to appeal because I was still too ill to go back to work.

I filed the appeals paperwork and waited for direction on what to do next. I learned that the social security disability department was behind on their caseload and I had a feeling that I was going to be waiting a while for a response from them. In February of 2008 Pat begin pressuring me to find out what was going on with my appeals so I called and spoke with the woman handling my case. She confirmed that they were still behind on their caseload. I shared the news with Pat and he became furious and began to shout at me that I wasn't doing enough and that I wasn't really sick, I was faking it because I just didn't want to work. Needless to say I was angry and hurt at his accusations. By this time I was totally fed up.

In May of 2008 I decided to contact the Caldwell and Ober law firm because their main focus was social security disability. Mark Caldwell agreed to take my case. I gave a plethora of information which included names, addresses, and phone numbers of endocrinologists, primary care physician, surgeons, ultra sound, thyroid scan uptake, x-ray technician, phlebotomist personnel along with the hospital information where both my Radioactive Iodine (RAI) therapy and total thyroidectomy were performed. Mr. Caldwell also needed dates all of the services rendered along with a list of medications and dates they had been prescribed. It was truly like having a job preparing all of this information. Finally all of the paperwork was filed and now we waited for a date to meet with an administrative law judge.

During this period of waiting, I received phone calls from Dan and he would often pray with me during our phone conversations. The prayers helped to keep the flicker of light from emerging from the cave in my vision as I remained hopeful that there would be light at the end of the tunnel. My brother, Pat, continued to come by to visit me and we would often reminisce about our times together growing up which always included laughter and fond memories of our parents and siblings.

Meanwhile, we continued to struggle financially trying to just keep up with our basic monthly living expenses. The financial stress was unbearable and we continually fought over the lack of finances. I hated to see the negative effect all of the stress and fighting had on my daughter Maria. Pat demanded that I e-mail Congressman Trent Franks to tell him of my plight. I received a phone call and a letter from the Honorable Trent Franks office assuring me that they had contacted social security disability on my behalf. Within days I received a letter from social security disability stating they were behind but would be looking at my appeals case within the next few months.

The one flicker of hope was that with Mr. Caldwell representing me my appeals had a better chance of being found favorable by the administrative law judge. This helped me to calm down as I waited for my appeals hearing.

Six months later, on December 10, 2008 my daughter and I drove (my Saab 9 3 Convertible was smoking from under the hood and I had to stop the car and pull over to a safe place to fill the coolant twice because it was leaking) to the Social Security Administration building. My hearing was scheduled for 9:15 am. Two years and 1 month after I initially filed for social security disability benefits I finally met with an administrative law judge, along with my attorney Mark Caldwell.

If you have filed for social security disability benefits and you have been waiting years for a favorable decision, I strongly encourage you to consider retaining legal counsel. Do not give up. I know that it is stressful to fill out all of the paperwork that is required. It took me several hours every time I had to complete the required paperwork. Sometimes I would literally cry out of frustration while filling out the forms because it was hard to remember the information that was requested. I also struggled with lack of focus (I still do) while attempting to prepare the paperwork. It was very difficult for me to pursue the disability benefits but it was necessary due to the intense financial strain we were experiencing. My husband was working full-time as a cashier as well as working long hours as a licensed realtor. Additionally, the financial pressure was putting a huge strain on our marriage.

I am thankful that I met with my attorney before the hearing. He counseled me and helped me prepare. My actual hearing lasted less than a half hour. After the hearing, Mark Caldwell and I met to review. He informed me that it would be weeks before we would hear the administrative law judge's decision.

As Maria and I walked into the elevator I began to cry. The pressure of having to wait so long for this day was finally gone. Maria and I hugged each other and prayed that God would grant us favor with the administrative law judge. On the way out of the building my daughter and I stopped to admire the beautifully decorated Christmas tree placed on the main floor. Now we could officially celebrate the Christmas holiday!

It was now January 10, 2009, a month after my appeals hearing and I began looking for the letter from the administrative law judge in hopes of a favorable reply. Days before my birthday, as I opened the mailbox and scanned quickly through the letters, I spotted a thick envelope with Social Security Administration typed in the return address portion of the envelope. I walked into the house, told Maria the letter was here and we went into the kitchen and sat down at the kitchen table. I quickly opened the letter and began to scan the contents. My eyes were drawn to the decision that I had been waiting for since November 5, 2006. Unfavorable.

I was extremely disappointed. I had no idea how we were going to go on financially. We had exhausted all of our financial resources and the commission money from the real estate sales had long been gone and used to pay our basic living expenses. I dreaded telling Pat that my appeal was denied. I had figured that with all of the back disability payments I would be getting a lump sum of approximately $18,000 from social security. I was also angry because I had always worked, ever since I was eighteen years old, and we desperately needed the money. I wasn't trying to pull a scam on the government. I was only trying to financially provide for my twelve-year-old daughter and alleviate some of the financial pressure from her father's shoulders.

Although the judge's ruling was a huge disappointment, to be truthful, I was relieved. Deep down I didn't want the label of being disabled. I wanted to return to my normal, healthy self. I wanted to be a positive contributor in the workforce. I wanted to use my God-given abilities and talents in a career. I didn't want this incurable disease to eliminate me from being gainfully employed.

I chose to trust God with this mountain of financial pressure. I chose to praise Him while I waited for an answer to our financial dilemma. I chose to take this setback and use it as a stepping stone as I continued to emerge from the cave.

Chapter Seven
Financial Pressures

My last day of full time work was June 9, 2006. We didn't have savings built up. Fortunately, Pat's employer, as a perk, paid our family medical insurance premiums. We were responsible for the doctors' visits, medical procedures and prescriptions co-pays, though. Additionally, an annual deductible must be met before we could take advantage of the percentage co-pays such as the hospital stay and actual total thyroidectomy.

Living on one income proved to be very challenging. The financial pressures became a point of contention with us. He resented the fact that I wasn't working and would regularly tell me that I was just faking it and that I wasn't sick. Further, I was just using it as an excuse to not work. These accusations deeply hurt me which caused problems to arise in other areas of our relationship. I would avoid him as much as possible because I abhorred his shouting at me and blaming me for our financial woes. I also didn't like Maria to hear the screaming and cursing that would come from his lips. I wanted to yell back at him and sometimes, due to complete exhaustion and utter frustration of living in the negative environment, I would yell at him. I hated what was happening. I never wanted to have an explosive marriage where the couples fought the majority of the time, yet this was exactly what was happening in the marriage. This was just another stressor to add to all of the other stressors in our lives.

The months dragged on and in 2008 I began to have to tap into our home equity line of credit to pay the mortgage, the property taxes, home insurance premium, all of the realtor fees, the medical co-pays and prescriptions, the utility bills and so on. Pat's income just didn't cover all of the living expenses that we had. The hospital co-pay for my total thyroidectomy was hundreds of dollars. A few weeks after my surgery we had another lean birthday party for Maria. I felt so guilty that I couldn't give her an amazing birthday bash like her other friends were having. I seemed to always feel guilty about something.

Then in the summer of 2008 we received a large check in the mail. It was Pat's inheritance from his mom, Carole. She lost her battle with lung cancer in February of 2007. We began to pay off credit card debts because we had been using credit cards to pay for our living and medical expenses. We still didn't have enough money to pay off the home equity line of credit. When Pat discovered that there wasn't enough money to pay that particularly large debt, he became furious and began to accuse me of stealing his mom's inheritance from him. He was vicious in his accusations verbally assaulting me and calling me vulgar names. All during our thirteen years of marriage I was very scared of these rages that he would go into. I felt defenseless because I was still recovering from my surgery, slowly, I might add. I felt humiliated and ashamed to be treated in such a fashion, especially by the very person who had promised to love, honor, and cherish me in sickness and in health. I would literally have a sick feeling in the pit of my stomach when Pat would go into these rages. I felt powerless and disgusted all at the same time. Our lives were spinning out of control due to financial pressures.

By 2009 the financial pressures were gripping us like a mighty vise. Even though Pat worked full time as a cashier, was a realtor and had made three sales in the latter part of 2008 we still continued to come up short. It was approaching one year since my total thyroidectomy but I had a myriad of health issues that were making it impossible for me to work full-time. We discussed the possibility of me going to real estate school and although I didn't want to, I reluctantly agreed. The reason that I agreed is because I thought that giving into Pat's insistence that I become a realtor would stop him from going into these rages against me over the financial pressures we had. Of course I was wrong.

In February of 2009 I enrolled in a two-week real estate salesperson crash course. I took notes while both of my eyes continually teared (a Graves' disease symptom) and the instructor noticed I was having problems with my eyes and asked if I was okay. I was on a fast track to total stress burnout but I couldn't get off now so I just did the best that I could.

After passing the school national and state exams, I failed the National Real Estate exam once and the State Real Estate Exam twice. This devastated me because I was a college graduate and yet was struggling to pass these real estate exams. I spent hours of studying but I wasn't studying effectively. Much to my embarrassment I sat in on a couple of the classes over again before I went back to take the State Exam the third time. It was on the third try that I successfully passed the State exam! After the proctor told me that I had passed the exam, I remember going into the bathroom at the testing center and literally sobbing for several minutes in thanks to God for finally passing the test.

Surely I thought this real estate accomplishment would please Pat because he had wanted me to become a realtor for years. I anticipated that he would now stop yelling at me, cursing at me, calling my filthy, vulgar names. As Maria and I were driving on the SR51 in my Saab 9 3 Convertible after leaving the AZ Dept of Real Estate, I felt that I was finally emerging out of life in the cave while listening to Jaci Velasquez sing "back into the light again". It was thrilling and exhilarating to feel that dark force growing dimmer and the light of hope and possibility becoming brighter as the wind whipped through our hair while we laughed and celebrated this important milestone.

That evening when Pat came home from work I excitedly told him I had passed the exam, drove straight over to the AZ Department of Real Estate to get registered, then went to his broker's office to sign up and I was now officially an active realtor. I asked him if we could go out to eat to celebrate. He yelled at me, called me a (insert inappropriate slang term) and told me he had worked all day long and he was too tired to go out. After he spent a while on the computer he went to bed. I don't even remember what Maria and I ate for dinner that evening.

The months went by slowly. The first six months of 2009 brought no financial relief. We were talking about the real possibility of losing our house in foreclosure. The arguments became more volatile. Pat would curse at me, scream at me, accuse me of stealing his mom's inheritance when he woke up, when he came home from work and even in the middle of the night he would wake me up yelling at me and start the whole cycle over again the next morning. Finally, early in June of 2009, I could no longer mentally or emotionally handle his rage and anger. I filed for divorce and Maria and I went into hiding. During this time I was working on my Final Edits for *Life in the Cave Overcoming Grave's Disease* at the hotel where we hid during the summer. This helped me to not slip back into utter despair. It was a task I desperately needed as I continued to emerge from the cave.

Maria and I bonded even closer as we enjoyed swimming in the pool, took Jett (Maria's Norwegian Forest cat) for walks, and dined in the onsite restaurant. We would linger at our table by the fountain in the evenings and as we listened to the water flowing in the fountain it relaxed us and healed our hearts. It was in these quiet moments that I would mediate on "Be still and know that I am God." Maria and I would smile at each other as we both felt the presence of the Lord with us. His light was with us while we were in hiding. He was giving us hope for a brighter future.

The brightness came to us as we became fast friends with both waitresses Donna and Phyllis. They consistently were kind to Maria. I appreciated the way they affirmed Maria by including her in conversations. I believe that God brought these two beautiful women into our lives to bring us light as we hid at the hotel.

Although we were in hiding, this moment in time continued the process of emerging from the cave. Maria and I had a glimpse of what our lives could be like surrounded by people who respected us and genuinely enjoyed our company.

Chapter Eight
Relationships

My first endocrinologist, Dr. Dolinar, informed us that many married couples divorce when one of the spouses has Graves' disease. He went on to say that the personality of the Graves' disease patient dramatically alters and the healthy partner sometimes can't deal with all of the personality changes. All I can share is that I was very irritable and the financial pressures aggravated all of the negative forces a million times over. I just knew that I had to get Maria and I to a safe place before we began to be physically harmed; we were already emotionally and mentally abused by Pat. Maria was not directly verbally abused but she still was a victim as she watched and listened in terror at the way her father was negatively treating her mother. Please keep in mind that we had a troubled marriage to begin with. If you are married it doesn't mean that you will wind up in divorce court. You need to be prepared to seek outside help, though, if serious problems arise that are not effectively resolved and you and your partner want to save your marriage.

By this time, the spring of 2009, I had no desire to reconcile with Pat. I didn't want to go to counseling. I didn't want to work on the marriage. I was done with this verbally abusive man who made me feel subhuman. I was a prisoner in my own home and I was very angry that I had stooped so low and unable to defend myself better. I was a college graduate, bright, talented and yet made to feel like the lowest of the lowest object on the planet. I hated Pat's behavior toward me and I hated myself for staying in this abusive relationship for so long. Back in the fall of 2001 I had planned to leave Pat and start a new life with my daughter. So once again, bear in mind, my marriage was troubled for nearly a decade before I finally filed for divorce and left in 2009.

This experience was another part of emerging from the cave. I slowly began to believe that I could remove myself from this subversive relationship in spite of the obstacles of not working full-time and battling an incurable disease. I welcomed this feeling of empowerment.

Your relationships with family, friends and the community are affected and normally change when you have Graves' disease. How close you are to family members, how often you see your friends and how active you are in the community will all yield different relationship results for every individual diagnosed with Graves' disease. The best that you can do is to provide awareness and education for those you are in relationship with in an effort to help them understand that it is the Graves' disease that is causing your personality to alter reminding them to not take your irritability personally. A suggestion would be for them to leave the area for a while and do a pleasant activity away from you when they can tell you are in a particularly foul mood. This gives you the space you need to get over it and the opportunity they need to refuel as well.

I strongly urge you to not to try to go it alone if you have Graves' disease. You need people in your life that sincerely love you and care about your wellbeing. You need to know that you are loved. You need that hug. You need that word of encouragement. You need to know that you matter. I appreciated the phone calls from my mom, my sister, and my brothers. My mom and sister also sent me thoughtful cards to brighten my days.

Open communication is what will save you in your relationships. You may want to consider individual counseling and family counseling if there are unhealthy ways of dealing with stress present in your closest of relationships. If you're still able to work I would suggest scheduling a meeting with your employer. It may be helpful to bring along Graves' disease articles to share that may help facilitate dialogue, education, empathy and understanding from your employer. Further, if your endocrinologist is open and available, ask if he/she would be willing to discuss Graves' disease with your employer providing an opportunity to gain knowledge about this disease from a medical professional.

You are in control of your relationships more than you realize. Even the best of relationships experience the ebb and flow of life and you need these meaningful relationships to get you through the dark days. An effective way to deal with your irritability and frustration is to journal those negative feelings you are experiencing in your relationships with others. Write them down. Read them. Vent them on paper. Then allow forgiveness to come from deep inside you for the offense and allow your love for that person to flow once again. Remember the ebb and flow and remind yourself of what drew you to that wonderful person in the first place.

You are forever changed and once you can accept that fact you will feel more empowered as you interact with others. Remember it is up to you to educate and stoke Graves' disease awareness in your relationships. Just as they need to be patient with you it is wise to remember that you need to be patient with them. You have changed and it will take time to adjust to these personality changes on everyone's part.

I challenge you to turn this deficit of irritability into an asset. You can do it. It will take effort and endurance while you all work through the necessary adjustments in your changed relationships. Don't give up, though. You will make it to the other side and look back to see how much closer and tighter your bonds are in these special relationships in your life. The joy that I've experienced in my relationships has continued the process of emerging from the cave and the light shines brighter each day.

As far as relationships in the community it varies for each person. Some of you may have been very active in your community and I challenge you to become a Graves' disease awareness activist in your circle of influence. There is a need for the world to know that Graves' disease is an autoimmune disorder that there is no cure for. It is a real disease with grave (no pun intended) results, for example, thyroid storm, where body temperature, blood pressure and heart rate all go sky-high, is life-threatening and could result in a stroke or heart attack if not treated properly. The patient must immediately go to the hospital to receive proper treatment for thyroid storm symptoms. Most people have never heard of Graves' disease. Let's change that fact and become the voice for those who have just been diagnosed and are too afraid, fatigued, overwhelmed and stressed to share their stories of their battle with Graves' disease. Let's be their voice until they are strong enough to speak up.

I have had family members, former coworkers, college friends and friends I've lost contact with over the years read my first book, *Life in the Cave Overcoming Grave's Disease* and call me (some even write to me) to apologize, even cry, because they weren't there for me. I don't have any ill will or grudges with these amazing people who have shaped my life. How could I when I didn't even understand what was happening to me before I was diagnosed? I do know that I now have an obligation to educate folks on Graves' disease as I've become stronger and am surviving Graves' disease.

In your relationships it is important to feel safe and also comforting to know you have support in these meaningful relationships. Support is key to surviving Graves' disease and the last chapter will explore this important topic.

Chapter Nine
Support

In closing, you must have support. Even if all you have is the support of one other person on the planet consider yourself rich. You cannot, I repeat, you cannot survive Graves' disease on your own. You need the support of others. A reader shared with me how she loved the title of my book *Life in the Cave* because that is exactly how she felt, like she was in a cave. It is so easy to believe the lie that you are on your own, that no one understands, that no one cares. Well, dear reader, I care. Folks who are members of and/or associated with the National Graves' Disease Foundation care, too. You are not alone. Even though only a small amount of the population has been diagnosed with Graves' disease each of us knows what it is like to feel overwhelmed with the many facets of Graves' disease and we are eager to stoke Graves' disease awareness.

In Chapter Eight I shared the importance of support in our relationships. Now I'd like to take a moment to look at online and local support groups.

There are many online Graves' disease discussion boards out in cyberspace. If you are a member of Facebook I personally invite you to join our Living with Grave's Disease facebook group at http://www.facebook.com/group.php?gid=231268090 678 There are other Graves' disease support groups on facebook, too. Another great place to go for online support, and in my opinion one of the best online resources, is http://www.ngdf.org

The National Graves' Disease Foundation has support groups in many states throughout the United States and in Canada. They are actively adding new support groups, too. Even if your state doesn't have a support group now the chances are good that it eventually will have one.

Lastly, I warmly invite you to email me at celiamarieauthor@gmail.com as I would love to hear your story. Please know that you are not alone in your battle with Graves' disease. I read each e-mail and personally answer every e-mail. Sometimes I do get behind on e-mails but I assure you that at some point you will hear directly from me.

Thank you for reading my story. It has been difficult to share some of the most intimate details of my life here with you but if it can help in some small way to aid you in surviving Graves' disease then it has been worth it.